WHAT IS HEALTHY COFFEE, AND HOW DOES GANODERMA LUCIDUM IN MY COFFEE MAKE IT HEALTHIER?

Petra Ortiz

Contents

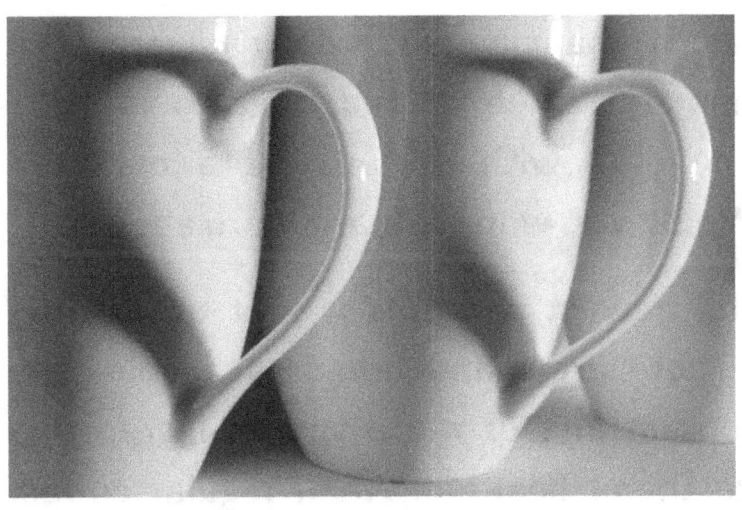

INTRODUCTION

Many people are concerned about how they appear to others, how attractive they are to a certain sex, how well they feel overall, how long they will live and also, how robust of a life they will be able to experience. A lot of them look to the internet for help. They search primarily for the easiest way to solve their problem(s). Some phrases they will type into a search engine field are 'quick and easy' ways to lose weight, increase stamina, decrease stress, fall asleep, stop smoking, stop snoring, stop worrying, save their marriage, find a date, and also many 'lower my risk of' [a variety of health] issues. What if by the simple act of changing your daily beverage of choice, namely coffee or tea, you could have positive benefits with one or more of those issues? Would you want to learn more about it?

One of the newest concepts is that of 'healthy coffee'. There are many brands available, and usually contain one or more special ingredients that make them 'healthier' than regular coffee. This book is meant to give information on one particular brand, which combines gourmet coffee with a very special ingredient. You will learn what that is, and how it has helped others. You will also learn how to consume it, what types of products are currently available, and a lot more. The main reason I created this book is so that you will have enough information to decide if it is something you are willing to try. It is my sincere hope that after you read this book, you will then take action and actually try 'healthy coffee'. Who knows, maybe you will decide you want to share this with others?

Throughout this book, you will find Coffee Scenarios which will give you additional information you may have never read or even heard about; and tips on how to share this coffee. I have also included options that can help save you a lot of time and money. In the last chapter, I will reveal to you how it has personally affected me, so that you know why I share it with others, and why this book is even available. Sprinkled throughout, you will find my personal recommendations on various aspects, plus advice and information that other caring and sincere people have shared with me.

Thank you for investing your time in learning about what I consider to be a Miracle in my life. I hope it can be one for you too.

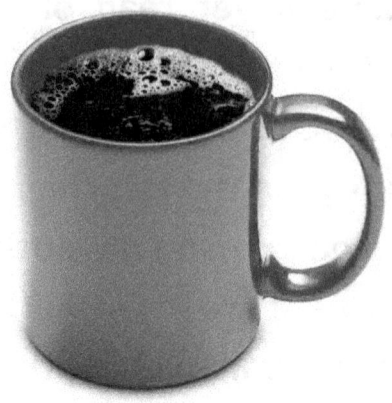

WHAT IS HEALTHY COFFEE?

Healthy Coffee IS coffee, first and foremost. This particular brand of gourmet coffee is 100% Arabica bean, and it is infused with a very special ingredient. Most people that have sampled this brand of gourmet coffee like or love the flavour. Most enjoy the aroma, and they notice and will comment on the exquisite taste; and they cannot believe it is 'instant' coffee. They also tell me that it doesn't taste 'bitter', and that they felt 'good' or 'great' after drinking it. Most people cannot taste, see, nor smell the 'health', all they say they experience is delicious gourmet coffee. Many notice that they do not run into the usual problems that occur while drinking 'regular' coffee. You probably know what I'm referring to:

jitters, crashing, burning stomach, acid indigestion, heart palpitations, nausea and the like. Most notice some kind of benefit too. The healthy beverages and supplements include Organic Coffee, Gourmet Coffee, Green Tea, Hot Chocolate, supplements and much more. Because of the special ingredient, these products can negate the effects of caffeine, and can positively affect your health. There are a multitude of coincidences that have occurred [a simple online search will reveal this to you]. It is helping many people across the Globe with various issues such as Diabetes, Black Mold, Carcinoid Tumors, PMS, Menopause, and more. You may want to do your own research to validate the power of this unique ingredient called Ganoderma Lucidum, for yourself. Currently, the wholesale price for the 'black coffee' version is just over 50 cents per serving, or cup, and about $1.00 per cup retail. So not only does it taste great, it is also competitively priced. And it can help YOU. It has positively affected me in so many ways [read my personal testimonial near the end], I can't help but tell everyone about this amazing coffee. I have saved a lot of money by using this brand for the past three years. If you decide to sample or buy this brand, you may want to start by drinking one cup per day. When you locate an Independent Representative [aka a Distributor] to mail or hand you a sample, make sure that you let him / her know how you liked the taste and how it made you feel.

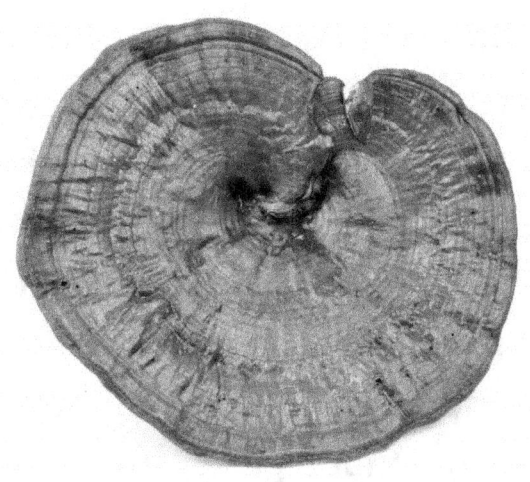

WHAT IS GANODERMA LUCIDUM?

Ganoderma Lucidum is a mushroom. A bright, shiny reddish-coloured mushroom. Ganoderma is often associated with longevity, youthfulness, and vitality. Ganoderma lucidum (also known as "Reishi" and "Lingzhi" in Japan and China, respectively) is found in nature, usually growing from hardwood deciduous trees such as maple and oak. The upper surface is a dark red colour, and so shiny, that it appears to be varnished. It is shaped like a giant fan, or kidney bean, and the cap can grow anywhere from 5 to 30 centimeters wide. The undersurface is tan to white in colour, and it has the appearance of suede. In nature,

Ganoderma Lucidum can be found growing (only two or three) out of every 10,000 aged deciduous trees [especially maple]. Emperors and kings valued it more than gold. Ganoderma has been known to be effective in the treatment of the widest range of health conditions. Unlike other mushrooms, only Ganoderma Lucidum has many important compounds such as triterpenes (ganoderic acid) that gives it its unique characteristic of being bitter in taste [remember, most people cannot detect any 'off' taste in this brand of healthy coffee]. Researchers have identified that water-soluble polysaccharides are one of the active ingredients found in Red Reishi, and that it has anti-tumor, immune modulating and blood pressure lowering effects. And studies have indicated that ganoderic acids help alleviate common allergies by inhibiting histamine release, improving oxygen utilization and liver functions.

I am not claiming healthy coffee is a cure for whatever ails you, or anyone else. But if you will just do your own research on Ganoderma [see my notes on 'how to'], you'll find that this mushroom is recognized as one of the most successfully used natural wellness ingredients, and it has been extensively studied in many clinical trials to document its curative properties. If you do a web search for 'Ganoderma' and any illness, you will find many web pages that will reveal what researchers, doctors and every day people have to say about this amazing substance.

Japanese researchers in the early 1970s discovered a method for cultivating it on a mass scale; it is now cultivated commercially in Japan, China, the US, and other parts of Asia. The processing plant for the world's leading brand of Ganoderma-based Healthy Beverages & Nutraceuticals is fully compliant with the USFDA Good Manufacturing Practice Standards (the highest in the world). The processing facility includes workshops for grinding, spore cell-wall breaking, mixing and making capsules, tablets, powder, and granule products. The advanced micro-particle milling [technology] is applied for the spore cell-wall breaking operation.

What does all this mean to you? It means you get the purest, highest quality, most bio-available version of Ganoderma, available anywhere at any price. This particular brand of healthy coffee is strategically infused with only 100% Certified Organic Ganoderma Lucidum. The purest form of Ganoderma Lucidum can be accessed directly from the Nutraceuticals, or supplements; especially for those who do not drink coffee, green tea nor hot chocolate. Ganoderma has been revered for over 5,000 years as the highest ranking "Superior Herb" in the ancient books of herbs and medicine. It is scientifically proven worldwide as nature's most potent health booster and overall conditioner. But like I said earlier, most people simply cannot detect it in this brand of healthy coffee- so have no fear...

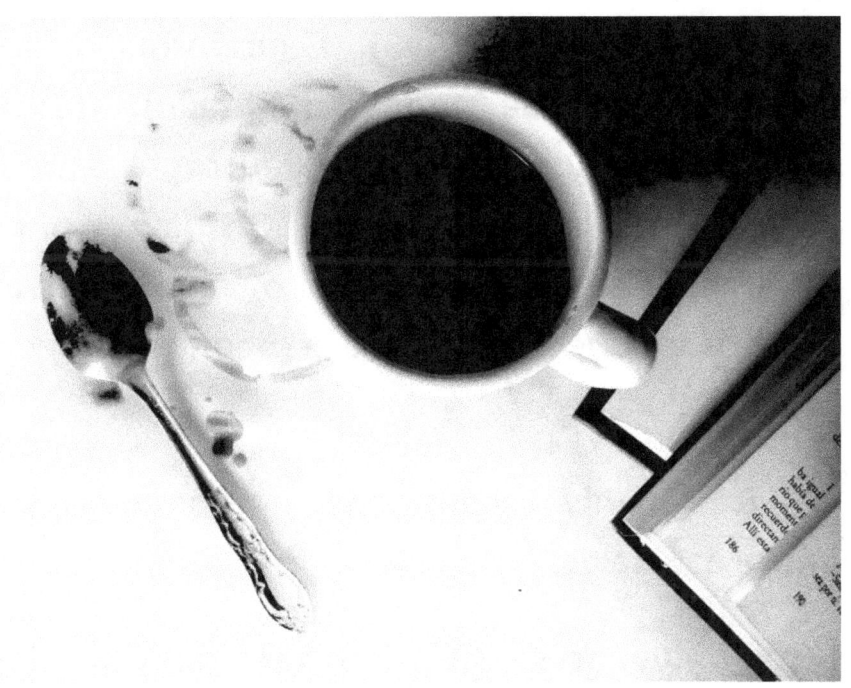

A Reishi Mushroom a Day May Keep the Doctor Away by Dr. Cathy Sabota, Horticulture Specialist

During the past 50 years, Asian countries have conducted an abundance of research on the medicinal value of several edible mushrooms. Their claims include reduction of blood pressure and cholesterol, enhancement of the immune system, cancer therapy, antiviral and anti-inflammatory properties, treatment of anaphylactic shock, anti-HIV properties, increase of oxygen utilization, and antioxidant properties

(Chen and Miles, 1996). Ganoderma lucidum (Reishi), Lentinula edodes (Shiitake), Hericium erinaceum (Lions Mane), Pleurotus ostreatus (Oyster mushroom), and Grifola frondosa (Maitake) are just a few of the cultivated mushroom species that have been analyzed for medicinal value.

NOTE: I highly recommend that you read the entire article at:

http://www.aces.edu/urban/metronews/vol3no 4/Mushroom.html

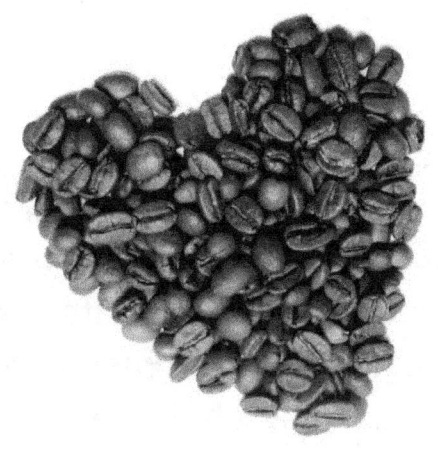

HOW HAS GANODERMA LUCIDUM HELPED OTHERS?

This particular brand of products is not intended to diagnose, treat, cure, prevent, or mitigate any disease and should never be offered as such. I do not suggest any diagnosis, prognosis, evaluation, treatment, description, management or remedy of illness, ailment or disease.

As a reminder, you should do your own research online for the particular issues that are of concern to you. You may want to visit any search engine online to see what I'm talking about; go ahead and type in:

'Ganoderma, heart disease'
'Ganoderma, arthritis'
'Ganoderma, diabetes'

Here is a brief list of issues that have coincidentally been affected by people around the world who have consumed Ganoderma Lucidum beverages and/or supplements [these include people I have personally sampled product to, and other people globally that I have read about in print, online, or watched on television or YouTube-you can do your own research any time]. There is no way to know for sure how it can affect a person, until they've actually consumed it:

blood pressure
cholesterol
dry eyes
watery eyes
sinus congestion
blood sugar
migraines
PMS
anxiety
overweight
arthritis
allergy symptoms

foot & leg swelling
energy
stamina
lactose intolerance
fibromyalgia
depression
acid indigestion
constipation
erectile dysfunction
irritable bowel syndrome

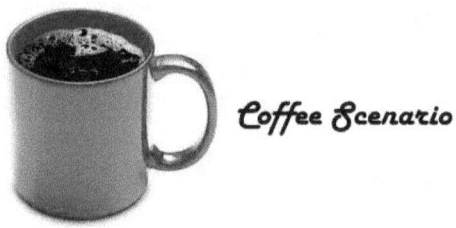

Coffee Scenario

COFFEE SCENARIO #1

Do you have access to hot water at work?

Bring your HEALTHY COFFEE sachets with you to the office, enjoy freshly prepared coffee for about $1.00 a cup Retail AND give yourself a boost.

Guess what happens next?

Your co-workers will ask about your coffee: you simply hand them some of yours to try...

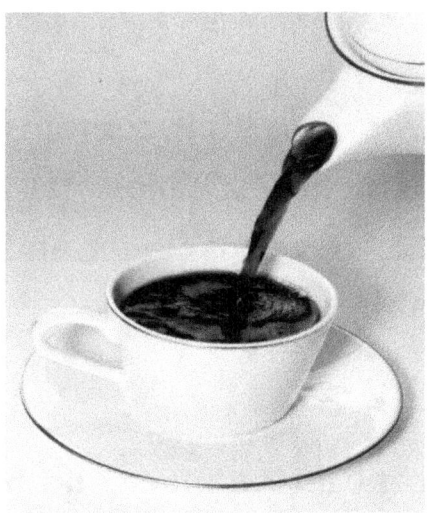

HOW DO I PREPARE IT?

[these are amounts I personally recommend-if it is too strong for you, just add water a bit more at a time]

GOURMET COFFEE BLACK

Empty contents of one sachet into a mug; Add 7 to 8 ounces of hot water. Stir. Enjoy. [add cream or cream and sugar as you normally would].

GOURMET LATTE OR MOCHA

Latte [includes creamer & sugar] or Mocha [includes creamer, sugar & chocolate] or Cafe Supreme. Empty contents of one sachet into a mug; Add 7 to 8 ounces of hot water. Stir. Enjoy.

ORGANIC GREEN TEA

Add 8 ounces hot water into mug that contains one teabag. Steep 2 to 3 minutes. Enjoy. [Or, steep 5 minutes, then add 2 to 3 cups water and chill to serve cold if you wish].

HOT CHOCOLATE

Empty contents of one sachet into a mug; Add 6 to 8 ounces of hot water. Stir. Enjoy.

ORGANIC KING OF COFFEE

Empty contents of one sachet into a mug; Add 7 to 8 ounces of hot water. Stir. Enjoy. [add cream or cream and sugar as you normally would].

ROYAL BREWED JAMAICA BLUE MOUNTAIN WITH GANODERMA SPORE

Place filter pack in your coffee maker [place it in the area where you would normally place a paper filter sleeve and add ground coffee to]. Add up to 18 ounces cold water to your coffee maker; turn 'on' - depending on your coffee maker instructions. Enjoy after completion of cycle.

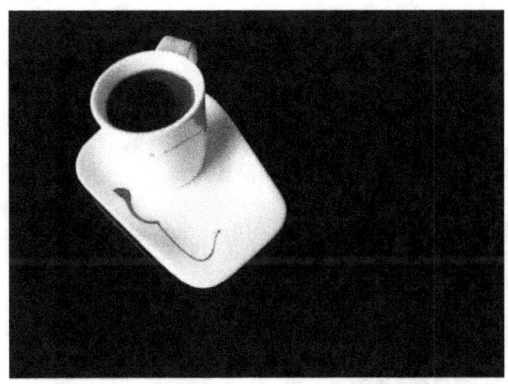

WHAT IS THE CAFFEINE CONTENT?

The caffeine in these products is naturally occurring. Naturally occurring caffeine can vary, depending on the variety of coffee or cacao beans, the blend and/or the brewing method.

- The caffeine in instant coffee ranges from approx. 60mg to 85mg per 8oz cup
- The range of caffeine in cocoa beverages is 3-32mg per 8oz. cup, with the typical being approx. 6mg

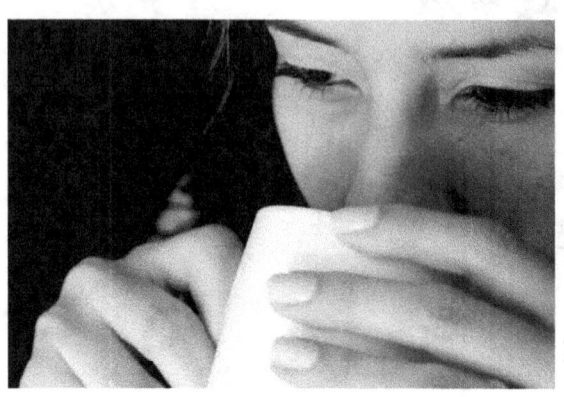

HOW CAN I LEARN MORE ABOUT GANODERMA LUCIDUM TESTIMONIALS?

You can do your own research online - head over to any search engine and type 'Ganoderma, ['any issue that concerns you']' or type 'Ganoderma testimonials' to find out how this 'King of Herbs' has helped many people around the world.

Locate an Independent Distributor online or in your local area, and ask for the issue of Health News issue on Ganoderma Lucidum testimonials. Don't forget to ask for a sample. In my opinion, if something tastes awful, I do not care how good it is for me-I won't consume it!

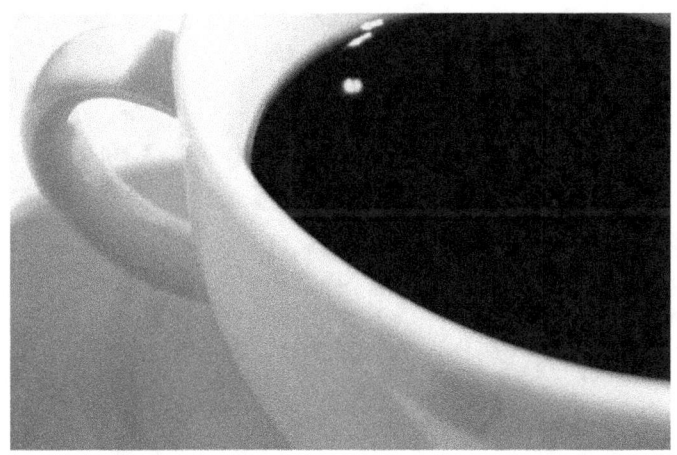

According to www.Reishi.com

A considerable number of studies in Japan, China, USA, and the UK in the past 30 years have shown that the consumption of red Reishi has been linked to the treatment of a vast range of diseases, common ailments, and conditions. From asthma to zoster, the applications of red Reishi seem to be related to a multitude of body organs and systems.

However, most of the scientific research that has been conducted appears to strongly support red Reishi's role as a normalizing substance - a nutritional supplement that can yield medical benefits through its normalization and regulation of the body's organs and functions.

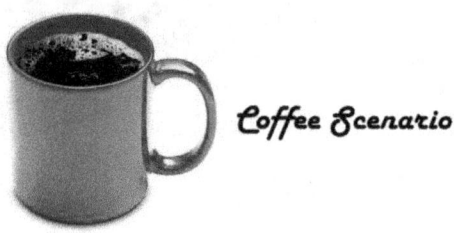

Coffee Scenario

COFFEE SCENARIO #2

You have already started consuming **HEALTHY COFFEE** on a regular basis, and have noticed a few benefits.

Why not share your personal testimony with your co-workers when they come sniffing around your office, asking what you are drinking...

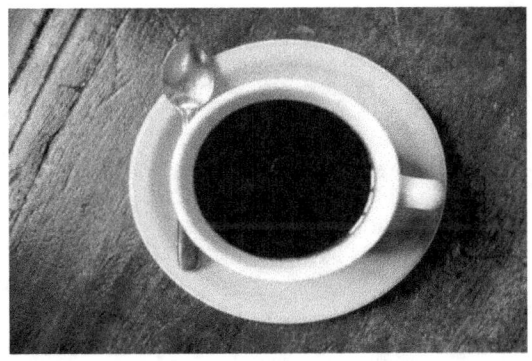

HOW MANY GANODERMA PRODUCTS ARE AVAILABLE?

There are several flavours of Coffee, an aromatic organic Green Tea, a Hot Chocolate, Skin Soap, and Toothpaste, plus pure form Supplements. Currently these are the items offered in the USA [however this brand is available in over thirteen countries and counting and new products are being formulated]:

BLACK/NOIR

This is Gourmet Black Coffee [high quality, aromatic Arabica remember?], most people that have sampled this flavour say it has a rich aroma and flavour, and they cannot believe it is from a sachet, rather than a freshly-brewed pot of coffee. There is no sugar in this flavour. It is packed in sachet form, 30 sachets in a box.

LATTE

This is Gourmet Black Coffee, with creamer and sugar included. Many people enjoy this one they say, because it is ultra-convenient for them: no need to carry creamer nor sugar packets with your coffee when on the go, traveling, commuting, at the office, etc. Packed in sachet form; 20 sachets in a box.

MOCHA

This is Gourmet Latte with the addition of the finest variety of Cocoa. People say this is like enjoying a rich and satisfying 'liquid dessert in a cup'. Packed in sachet form; 15 sachets in a box.

KING OF COFFEE

This is Organic Gourmet Coffee, with the addition of 100% Certified Organic Ganoderma Spore Powder. In my personal opinion, this is the best tasting gourmet healthy coffee flavour, and I feel very happy within 20 minutes of my first cup. It has a different flavour than the Black/Noir. To me it is reminiscent of mild flavours of cocoa, coconut, and nuts. For you, it could taste totally different. You should definitely try this one. Packed in sachet form; 25 sachets in a box.

ROYAL BREWED JAMAICA BLUE MOUNTAIN

Brewable Coffee with Ganoderma Spore. This is Premium Gourmet Royal Brewed utilizing the brand 'Jamaica Blue Mountain' Coffee, and infused with 100% Certified Organic Ganoderma Spore Powder. Packed in 'filter brew packs' for coffee maker utilization. Each filter pack makes about 18 ounces of coffee [3 six ounce cups] depending on the strength you like. 10 filter packs in a box.

CAFE SUPREME

Gourmet Latte featuring the superior Panax Ginseng plant [which was considered an herb of such great value in the ancient world that it was only available to people of great power and privilege- it is still highly prized and treasured in Asia as a key source of health and well-being]. It combines the power of Ginseng and 100%

Certified Organic Ganoderma, for a smooth 'perfect' blend. Packed in sachet form; 20 sachets in a box.

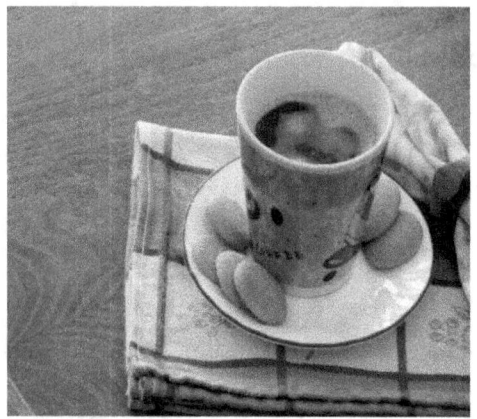

HOT CHOCOLATE

This is a Cocoa beverage [not coffee]. This is a Gourmet Hot Chocolate beverage, packed with the goodness of Ganoderma, just like all the other products. My younger sons look forward to drinking this beverage, and even though they don't 'tell me' it makes them feel great-as a Mom, I can tell that they are noticeably happier and more calm at the same time. Packed in sachet form, 15 sachets in a box.

ORGANIC GREEN TEA

This is Organic Green Tea [not coffee]. In my opinion, it has a lovely aroma and if I feel I need extra help falling asleep-this does it for me. You can enjoy it hot or cold. You may like it in one cup, or up to 3 or 4 cups, depending on how you like your green tea flavour: stronger or milder. I enjoy it iced as well [I dilute one steeped cup in 3 more cups of water then chill and enjoy iced & sugared throughout the day during warmer weather]. Packed in teabag form; 25 teabags in a box.

PREMIUM SKIN SOAP

It is a unique combination of Glutathione, Grape seed and Ganoderma Lucidum Extract. Its special formulation cleanses, moisturizes, and is hypoallergenic. Regular use promotes skin's youthful vibrancy. It can lighten and moisturize the skin, and prevent skin allergies and pigmentation. NOTE: The first time I used it on my face, my skin seemed to peel off 'old dead skin'; by the 2nd and 3rd use, my skin felt wonderfully soft [and no peeling] and I, and others that have used this soap, receive compliments on our 'glowing' complexion. Packed as a 4.76 ounce bar in a sealed box; 3 bars in a package. Sample sizes available.

TOOTHPASTE

A toothpaste with 100% Organic Ganoderma and the fresh taste of mild mint developed for the special care of your teeth and gums. It contains natural products that promote oral health and leave you with whiter teeth and fresher breath. My favourite ingredient is Honeysuckle- it gives this toothpaste an interesting flavour, an amber-like colour, and a nice mild 'honey-like' fragrance. It is very pleasing to me. 150 grams in a tube; packed one tube in a box. Sample sizes available.

GANODERMA LUCIDUM EXTRACT SUPPLEMENT

This is 100% Certified Organic Ganoderma Extract; a potent health booster and overall conditioner. Ganoderma is often associated with longevity, youthfulness, and vitality. Packed in capsule form; 90 capsules in a bottle.

GANODERMA MYCELIUM EXTRACT SUPPLEMENT

This is extracted from an 18-day old Ganoderma Lucidum mushroom with a naturally high concentration of Organic Germanium and Polysaccharides. Ganoderma Mycelium is also known to promote healthy circulation and oxygen supply; it is an immune system enhancer. Packed in capsule form; 90 capsules in a bottle.

GANODERMA SPORE EXTRACT SUPPLEMENT

Spore Powder is derived from the seeds of Ganoderma Lucidum. Carefully harvested, the spore contains the most nutritionally dense and bioavailable form of Ganoderma. It is cultivated from natural log wood, extracted through low-temperature shell-broken technology [reaching as high as 99.9% purity] and Certified Organic by China, USA, Japan, and the E.U. The Spore Powder is naturally rich in Ganoderma Lucidum Polysaccharides, Triterpenes, Organic Germanium and Selenium. Packed in capsule form; 90

capsules in a bottle. I personally open a capsule and empty the contents into my cup of healthy coffee, for an extra 'lift'. I cannot personally detect any difference in the taste of my coffee after mixing this one in. This is my favourite form of Ganoderma!

GRAPESEED OIL EXTRACT SUPPLEMENT

Does not contain Ganoderma. This supplement is pressed grape seed oil and yields a treasure trove of antioxidants and essential fatty acids; it is composed of phytochemicals known for their anti-inflammatory action, free radical protection and improving skin tone. It incorporates significant amounts of resveratrol [another substance that acts as an anti-inflammatory agent]. It also includes flavonoids or Oligomeric Procyanidins (OPCs), which are known to have 50 times more potent anti-oxidant protection than other Vitamin C or Vitamin E. Packed in encapsulated form; 30 capsules in a bottle. Search online to learn more about OPCs.

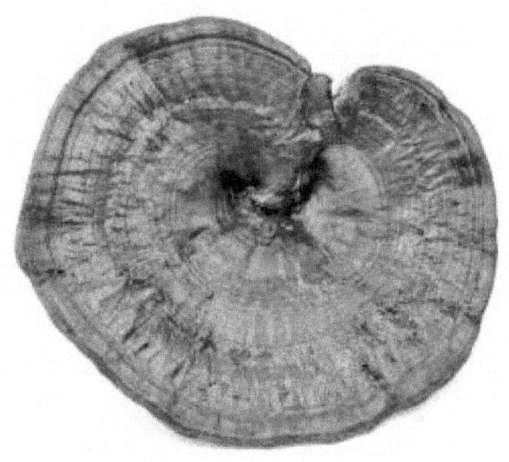

HOW DO I CONSUME GANODERMA SUPPLEMENTS?

As with any new treatment or even exercise regimen, I highly recommend that you discuss this with your doctor before deciding to take any course of treatment.

Some people start out by consuming one capsule per day, for up to 7 days. Depending on how they feel the first couple of days, will govern how many they believe they should consume. This is applicable to any of the capsules. [I dislike swallowing capsules or any types of pills, or tablets, because after my accident I was prescribed several medications and most were in

'big pill or capsule' form. So rather than swallow a capsule, I can easily open one Ganoderma Spore powder capsule into my coffee on days when I feel I will need extra energy.]

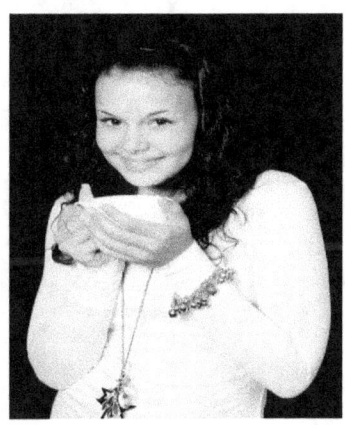

HOW DO I LEARN MORE ABOUT THIS BRAND OF HEALTHY BEVERAGES AND SUPPLEMENTS?

Locate an Independent Distributor online or in your local area [check the end of this book to find out what brand this is]. Ask them to send you a product sample, and a video overview [via email or website URL] for you to watch from your home. Within 24 to 48 hours of consuming the sample beverage, contact that Distributor and let them know

[1.] How you liked the taste.

[2.] How it made you feel (the day that you consumed it).

Ask them for a Health News issue on Ganoderma Lucidum to learn how it has helped many people around the world.

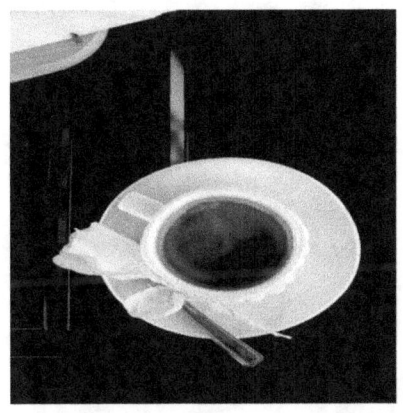

According to Wikipedia the largest online encyclopedia:

Numerous studies of lingzhi, mainly in China, Korea, Japan and the United States, have shown its effectiveness in the treatment of a very wide range of diseases and symptoms. But the studies have not given any explanation of exactly how lingzhi (Ganoderma) has so many diverse effects, because none of the known active components taken alone have produced results as powerful as the intake of lingzhi itself, suggesting synergy is important. For example, reports of lingzhi's effect on stamina, appetite, and other human conditions are largely anecdotal and haven't been studied scientifically. It is perhaps more comprehensible at this time to explain lingzhi's "miraculous powers" from the traditional Chinese medicine point of view.

Reference: Wikipedia.org

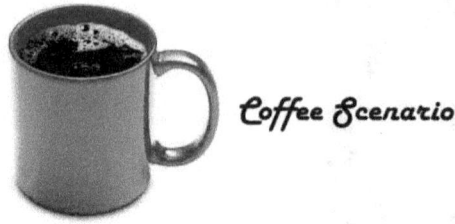

Coffee Scenario

COFFEE SCENARIO #3

Have you read a HEALTH NEWS issue on Ganoderma Lucidum yet?

Ask your chosen Distributor for a copy. Read the testimonials, and anytime that you happen to overhear someone mention an issue you read about in the Health news issue, tell them what you learned, then consider sharing your HEALTHY COFFEE with them.

Remember to ask them how they liked the taste and how it made them feel!

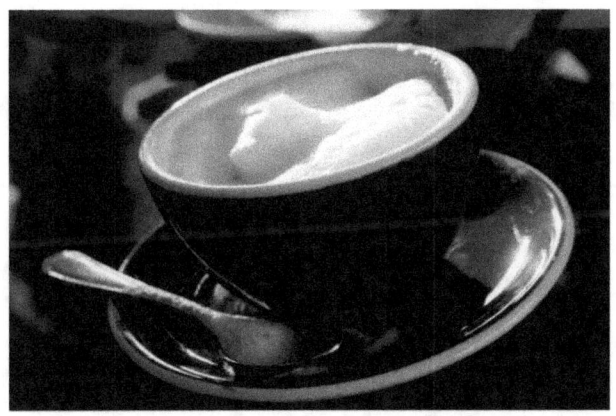

HOW DO I LISTEN TO A LIVE OVERVIEW?

You may want to learn about this brand in person, at a live event in your area. Locate an Independent Distributor online or in your local area. Ask them to give you a formal invitation to a Coffee Jazz Mixer, or any Coffee Tasting event that is taking place in your local area. You will probably have fun at this event.

Additionally, you can always visit the Distributor's website and click EVENTS to see what mixers will be in your area.

Make sure that you arrive on time, sample the products you are interested in, take notes and then ask your chosen Distributor any questions you have about this brand.

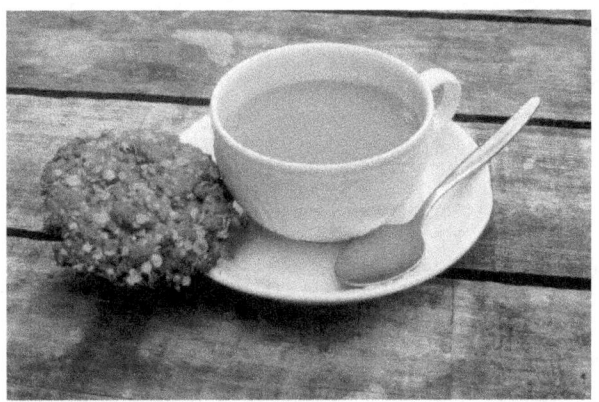

WHAT IS A COFFEE BREAK CALL?

You may want to learn more about this brand by listening to a phone call. A Coffee Break call is a live call aired daily, usually around 10:30am CST, meant to relay product health testimonials. Ask your local Distributor for the phone number, and pin code to listen live. You will want to have a notepad and pen handy in case you want to jot pertinent information down. There are recorded Coffee Break Calls available online as well. Ask your Independent Distributor for this information.

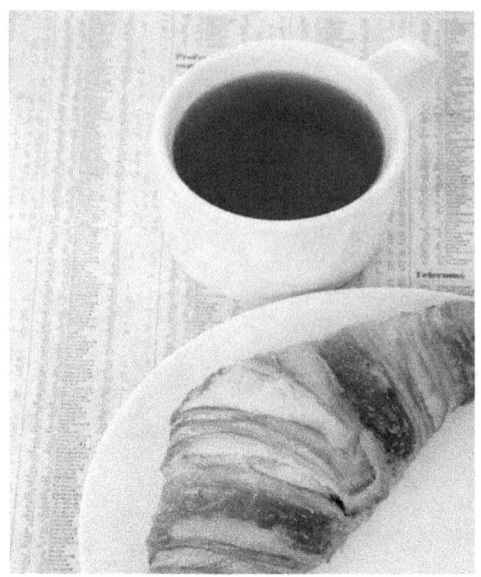

WHAT IS A CJM?

You may want to experience this brand 'live' with other coffee lovers. 'CJM' is an acronym for Coffee Jazz Mixer. It is a combination coffee-tasting event & product overview presentation; usually with jazz music playing for ambience. All guests are welcome to sample coffees and other beverages, read information about the products and testimonials, mix and mingle with other coffee lovers, then, after a short while they are introduced to a live overview or shown a DVD or video presentation that covers coffee in general, the healthy coffee beverages, information about

Ganoderma Lucidum and its benefits, and the opportunity available for retail or wholesale purchase, plus distribution options. Consumers are welcomed to give their own personal testimonials if they wish to do so.

There is usually a question & answer session. Guests are able to become retail or wholesale customers, or even Independent Distributors [to share the products and earn income for sales of products] if they choose to do so at the end of the event.

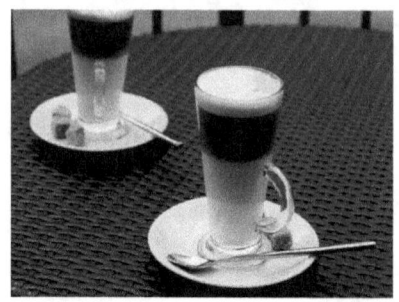

HOW DO I HOST MY OWN CJM?

Hosting a CJM [Coffee Jazz Mixer] is loosely described here. It is best to ask your Local Distributor for assistance on hosting your first four CJMs for best results. This would generally be undertaken if one decides to become an Independent Distributor:

1. Receive Guests and have them make their desired flavour(s) of coffee, tea, hot chocolate. {Jazz Music playing!}
2. Invite them to watch a Product & Customer Overview presentation. This is either a live presenter, a DVD presentation, or both.
3. Have a short Q&A [question and answer] session.
4. Complete any paperwork for those who wish to become wholesale customers or

Independent Distributors. Allow guests to leave.

5. Provide a brief Training session for all Independent Distributors & scheduling of new CJMs.

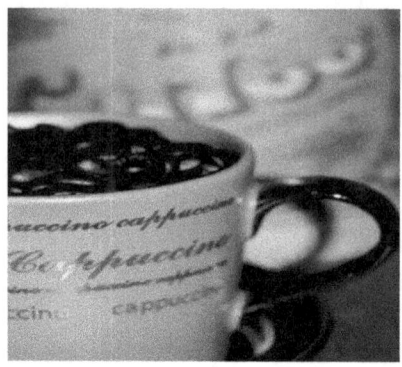

HOW DO I BECOME A WHOLESALE CUSTOMER?

You may want to buy the product at wholesale pricing shortly after you've sampled it. Or, you may decide that you like or love this product so much, that you'd rather spend less money when you buy it [after you've consumed one or two boxes]. In either case, you will want to locate an Independent Distributor online or in your local area and ask about becoming a Wholesale Customer. You have two options: you can click the JOIN NOW button at that Distributor's company-provided website, or complete an application and hand it to your local Distributor so he/she can manually add your website & system setup. It only takes a few minutes to complete the online process, and you will receive a 'welcome' email with your own company-provided website that will allow you to place your orders anytime you wish, but pay wholesale prices, rather than retail. The membership lasts for one full year. Additional year membership is available at a really amazing discounted price, and a reminder populates when you log into your site, in case you wish to renew, about two weeks before. Shipping is via UPS, and starts at $5.00 USD for one box, and increases slightly for additional boxes in each order. Make sure to ask the Distributor for assistance if you need it, when ordering. Read the chapter on instructions to place a wholesale order.

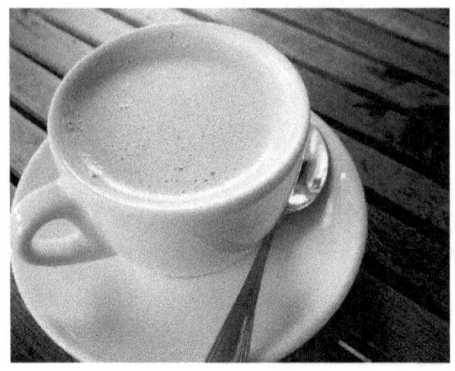

HOW DO I BECOME A RETAIL CUSTOMER?

You may want to buy one or two boxes immediately, at Retail price, to begin enjoying this brand of healthy coffee. To do that, you should locate an Independent Distributor online or in your local area. You have two options. You can order directly from that Distributor, and he/she will deliver the product(s) or meet you somewhere to deliver the product(s) or, You will need to ask them for their website URL [their link, so you can visit online]. You can attend a CJM and buy it Retail there.

At their website, you will need to click BUY PRODUCTS, choose the country you are in [currently only three are available in this particular section: USA, CANADA, and JAMAICA].

You will then click 'beverages, nutraceuticals, or skin care', choose the items you desire; click ADD TO CART, complete your purchase. You will receive your items via UPS. Currently the price for shipping one box is $5.00 USD, and increases slightly for additional boxes in each order.

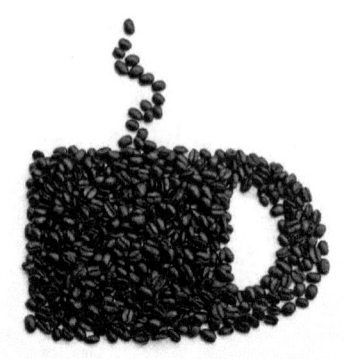

HOW DO I PURCHASE PRODUCTS AS A NON PROFIT ORGANIZATION FOR FUNDRAISING PURPOSES?

Locate an Independent Distributor online or in your local area. Ask for a Non-Profit/Health Care Practitioner Application. Read it completely. If you decide to complete the application, contact your chosen Distributor for assistance and processing. He/She will need to send it to the company for approval. Upon approval, ask your Distributor for the PDF file of the 'Order Form'. This can be used to accept orders for your fundraising event(s). Currently the first year Fundraising application fee is waived for non-profit organizations. Additionally, with a minimum purchase per order, shipping charges are waived. Ask your Distributor about these issues for clarification. This type of fundraiser allows for the opportunity to raise funds for one's cause each and every month, as coffee drinkers generally drink all year long.

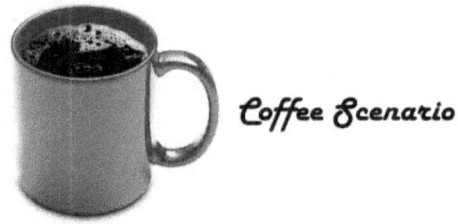

Coffee Scenario

COFFEE SCENARIO #4

For Organizations that utilize this brand of healthy coffee products to raise funds, there is a ready-made PDF Order Form available.

Log into your company provided website for a Document labeled ORDER FORM for Organizations.

All they have to do is print it and photocopy it, or print several forms; and then hand it to their members each month for order-taking purposes.

Or, you can design your own form!

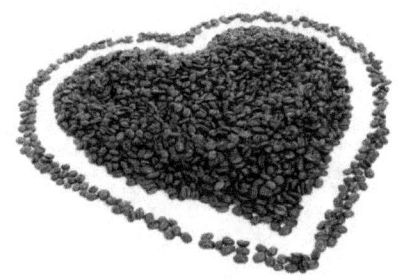

HOW DO I PURCHASE PRODUCTS AS A 'FOR PROFIT' ORGANIZATION FOR FUNDRAISING?

Locate an Independent Distributor online or in your local area. Ask for a Application for Distribution. As with any wholesale customer or Distributor, you will pay the initial first year Distributorship fee. Ask your Distributor for clarification on this. You will need to complete an application and furnish it to your chosen Distributor for submission to the company [and for approval].

Your chosen Distributor should assist you with how to use the Order Form, and how to submit your orders.

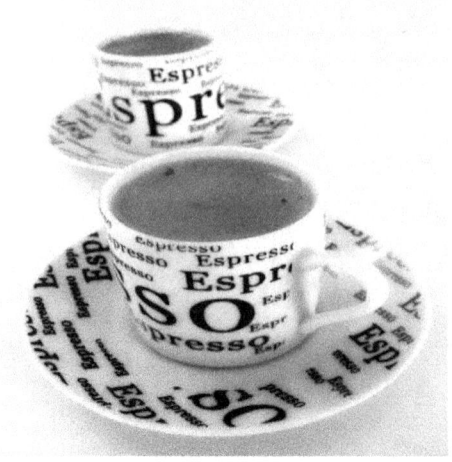

HOW CAN I SHARE THE PRODUCT TO EARN INCOME?

Ask your chosen Distributor for assistance and clarification. This would be something that an Independent Distributor would do to introduce products to the community to generate Retail and Wholesale customers:

Basically, ensure you are a product of the product, share your testimonial and sample products to others on a continuous basis. Hosting [or Inviting to] CJMs, attending training events as your Distributor instructs. After watching an Overview presentation, you will also have a better understanding of how to qualify to earn income. The sale of products is what effects commission earnings.

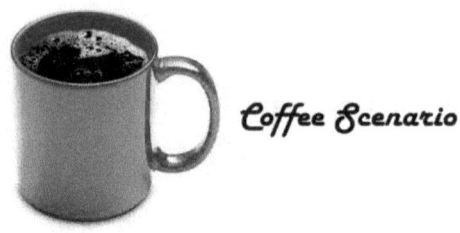

Coffee Scenario

COFFEE SCENARIO #5

Here are some ways you can generate Retail Sales of your HEALTHY COFFEE...

Beauty Salons & Spas

Person to Person

Fundraising Organizations

Barber Shops

Gyms

Fitness Centers

Health Care Practitioners

Consumer Shows

Festivals

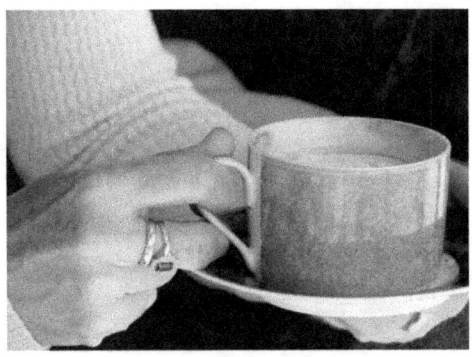

HOW CAN I DRINK THE PRODUCT TO EARN INCOME?

See previous chapter too. Again, this is only for those who wish to share the product(s), to sell products and earn additional income as an Independent Distributor so: ask your chosen Distributor for clarification and assistance, including an overview of the compensation plan. There are short and more in-depth videos and information available to clarify this for you.

Basically, as you are purchasing product at wholesale pricing, for your own [and your family's] personal consumption; learn how to qualify to earn income. The sale of products, produces commission earnings. Learn the 4 Steps and Learn the 4 Questions To Ask.

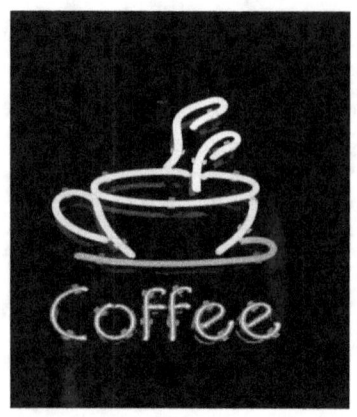

HOW DO I 'SIGN SOMEONE UP' TO MY GROUP OF CUSTOMERS AND DISTRIBUTORS?

First of all, you should always ask your chosen Distributor for assistance. In the event you are unable to receive assistance in a timely manner, here is a brief instruction set:

1. You can send your company website URL to your prospective customer / distributor and ask them to click the JOIN NOW link and enter their application online in that manner.

2. They can furnish a completed application to you [the application is in your back office: log into your company provided website], and you will add them 'manually' when you log into your company-provided

website. You would click DUAL TEAM VIEWER, to choose the team you want to place that person into- your left team or right team. After you have chosen which team, you are then presented with the same screen that your prospective wholesale customer or distributor would see when they click JOIN NOW choose their country and they then proceed from there.

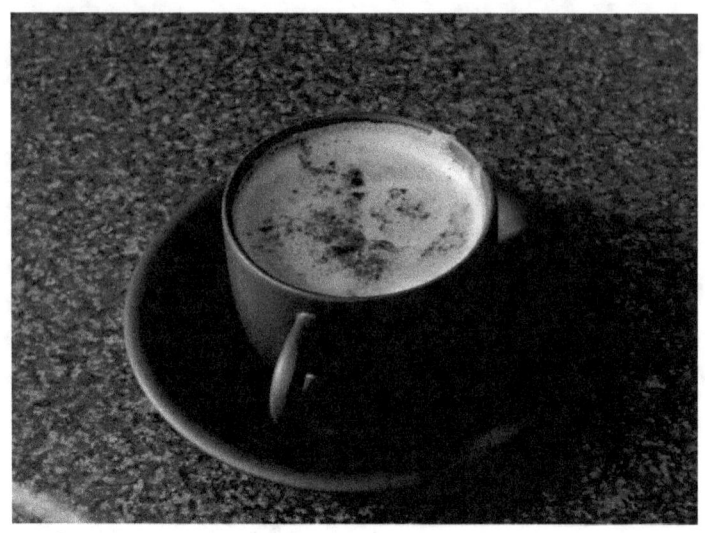

HOW DO I PLACE A WHOLESALE ORDER?

If you decide to buy [any of the] products wholesale, you have purchased a one year membership and are now considered a Wholesale Customer.

You will need to log into your company-provided website and click LOG IN. Enter your ID # or Username, then your password and 'enter'. You will click SHOPPING CART on the left side of your screen, and proceed from there; order your products and select desired quantities. Enter your billing and shipping information. You will have the opportunity to print your order after submission. It will also be available for viewing and printing whenever you log into your company-provided website. Alternatively, you can print [from your logged in state look for COMPANY DOCUMENTS, then 'ORDER FORM'] an ORDER FORM, complete it, then FAX IT to the Company for processing. Your order will arrive via UPS [United Parcel Service].

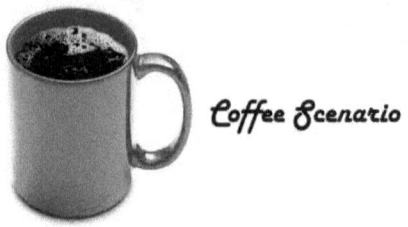

Coffee Scenario

COFFEE SCENARIO #6

If you want to make sure you always have enough coffee on hand for:

Your own Personal Consumption
Your Retail Customers
Your Sampling for the Month
Your Wholesale Team Partners
Your New Retail Customer Sales

You will want to ask your Sponsor how to get setup for the Autoship program. You designate the products and quantities of each, and then you designate the 1st or the 15th of the month to ship the items to you. The credit card you designate for Autoship is charged on the same day they are shipped. Note: if you need to modify your order that is on record for Autoship-you simply delete that 'order', and create a brand new one.

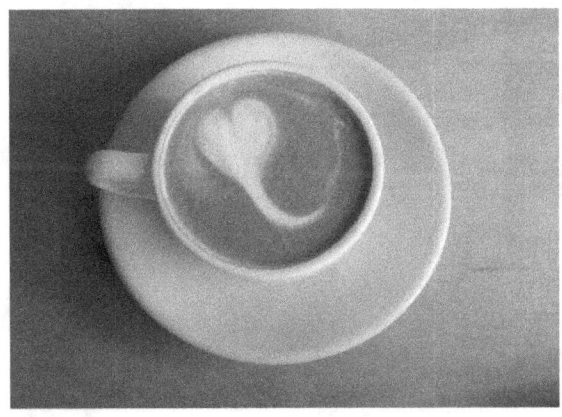

WILL I HAVE A 'COFFEE SCRIPT' TO FOLLOW FOR ORDER TAKING?

Yes. The first way you should set out finding customers is to use a Coffee Script. Ask your chosen Distributor / Sponsor for a copy of the Coffee Script to pre-sell your coffee products & officially launch your business.

It is a simple straightforward script meant to verbalize to your closest friends and family [you know, the people who should be willing to support your business launch] that you are starting a new endeavour and you appreciate their support. See the COFFEE SCENARIO #8 for an example Coffee Script.

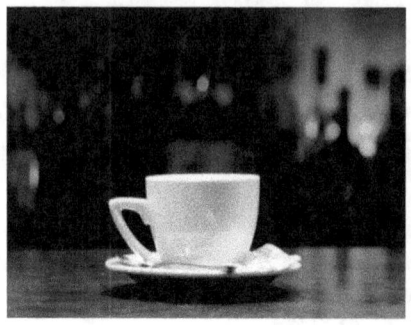

HOW DO I TAKE ORDERS VIA PHONE?

When you receive an order for product via a phone call, you should ask for the following:

1. Full Name
2. Phone Number
3. Address
4. Ask how they will pay for their order [decide what types of payment you will accept]
5. Decide on how you will get the order to the Customer: Deliver, Pickup, etc.
6. Let them know what day they can expect to receive their order [if you don't have the particular items in your inventory at the moment]

It is a great idea to let all your Retail Customers know, when you will be receiving orders and payments. For example: you can let them know that you will be accepting orders the last week of each month, for delivery the following month. You may want to schedule a lineup of phone calls that week to ask for their orders; many people are busy and will appreciate you taking the time to remind them not to miss out on this valuable product. *It is no fun to be without this coffee!*

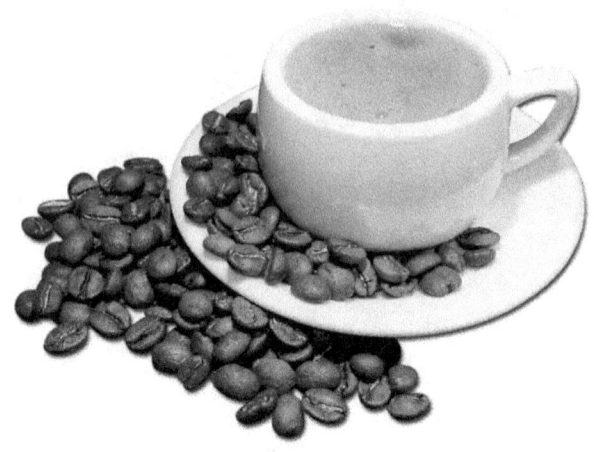

HOW DO I TAKE ORDERS VIA MY WEBSITE?

Your website, blog, ads are available 24/7 for anyone searching online, so even if you are on vacation, sleeping or lunching-it's possible for anyone to place an order for your product(s). But it is better for you to actively promote your sites. I mention just two options here, but you have more:

If you are utilizing the optional coffee marketing system [I call it the CM system] for online promotion and order-taking, visitors will order on that website of yours [they will order from your 'Retail Center' page]; payment is accepted via PayPal [they pay for their product using their

PayPal funds or their credit card-make sure you have a Premier Paypal account setup – it's free to do], and you are sent an email notification of the person's order. You will then need to deliver or mail the products, from your own inventory of products. It is a good idea to send the customer an email acknowledgement of their order, and when they can expect to receive it. If you use USPS [United States Postal Service] you may want to get 'delivery confirmation' for an extra charge to ensure the day, date and time your items were delivered to your customer. Ask your chosen Distributor for clarification on the profit margin.

If someone orders product directly from your company-provided website [meaning, they clicked BUY PRODUCTS, and ordered in this manner], the company receives the order, collects their payment via credit card, ships the products directly to the customer's shipping address; and sends you a check for the difference [retail minus wholesale price]. Ask your chosen Distributor for clarification on this matter.

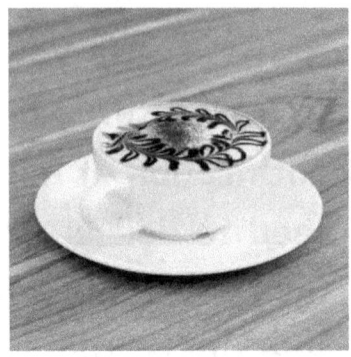

HOW DO I ENTER A PERSON'S ORDER 'IN PERSON'?

For a verbal or phone order: Write down [a good idea: have a receipt book handy at all times] the person's name, address, items ordered, individual prices, total amount due, and how the customer pre-paid for the order (via check, credit card information, cash).

Let them know when they can expect to receive a call from you for delivery OR when they can expect to receive a call from you for them to pick up-depending on the relationship you have with this customer. If you have the products ordered on hand [in your personal inventory] you can simply deliver the items when ordered.

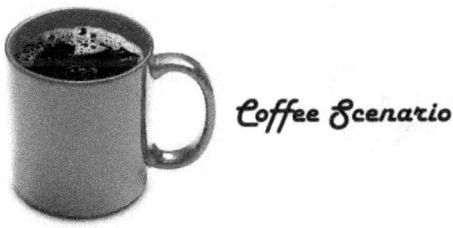

Coffee Scenario

COFFEE SCENARIO #7

Thank your customer for their order, and ask them to share their testimonial with others so that they can direct more prospective customers your way.

Bring them extra HEALTH NEWS issues with your contact information labeled on each one, then ask them to share the issues with those they care about.

Tell them you will be happy to give their referrals a free sample too, and make sure to bring your established customer product samples.

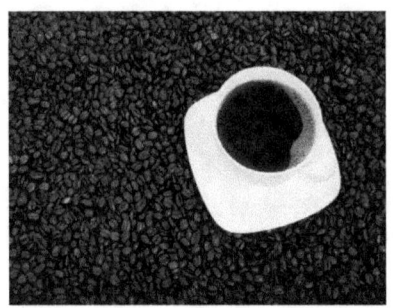

HOW DO I ENTER A PERSON IN MY GROUP ON MY LEFT OR RIGHT TEAM?

If you wish to become a **Wholesale Customer** or a **Distributor**, you will need to have your chosen Distributor [your Sponsor] assign your membership. For a Distributor, this is one of the ways to earn income with this brand of healthy coffee, by referring new customers. The default system is setup to place one person on the Left side, then the next person on the Right side [when they click **JOIN NOW** at your company provided website] and so on. But, briefly:

1. Log into your company-provided website
2. Click **DUAL TEAM VIEWER** [on the left side of the screen]

3. Choose [click] 'extreme outside left' or 'extreme outside right'
4. Select the symbol that corresponds with an 'open' position in your organization

Proceed from there with either the application in hand, or the person in your presence to complete the information.

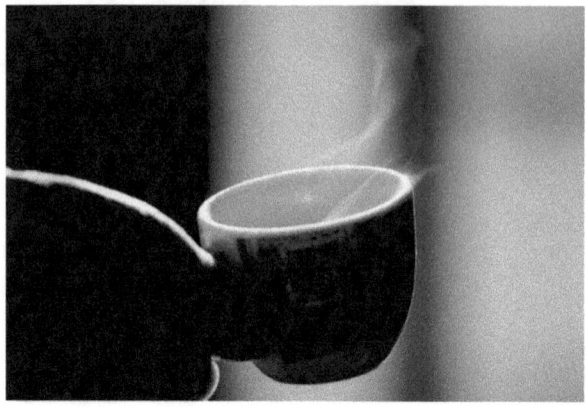

HOW DO I TRAIN A NEW DISTRIBUTOR ON MY TEAM?

Ask your chosen Distributor for help on this matter [your Sponsor], but briefly:

Follow the 4 STEPS TO SUCCESS

Learn how to ASK THE 4 QUESTIONS

Schedule CJMs [you should schedule these immediately] on a regular basis.

'Plug In' to the system

Your Sponsor will teach you how to plug in to they system, how to help your customers, how to order products, pre-sell using the Coffee Script, and show you how to invest your time more wisely and efficiently to help you achieve your goals.   Do enjoy helping people feel better? Are you able to follow directions and are you willing to invest your time in productive activities, to help you get what you want?

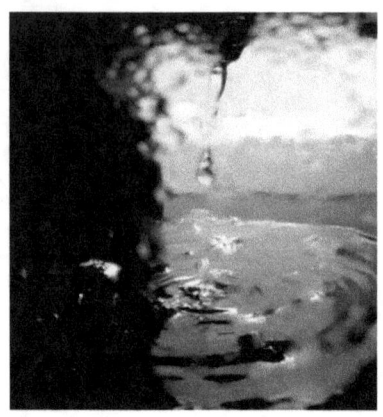

HOW DO I PROMOTE MY HEALTHY COFFEE PRODUCTS ONLINE?

A Distributor has several options, one that I personally value the most is an optional marketing system I affectionately call 'the CM SYSTEM'.

The following is my personal review of this system: When I first started using it over 2 years ago, I had very good results if you consider the number of leads opting in. The system sends the online prospective customer to an entertaining but concise video; beneath the video is a photo of the Distributor along with a message about the products and the opportunity in sharing them. A survey beneath the message allows the

Distributor to determine if the prospect (that has completed it) is interested in learning about the opportunity to earn income by drinking and sharing the products, or, just interested in consuming the products for their own personal benefit. There are several lead capture pages, and movie lead capture pages [a lead capture page is a website a person visits that offers information in exchange for the visitor's name and email address; he/she then receives the information in their inbox and they may be sent instantly to a site with an informative video to watch].

If a Distributor speaks to someone in person, that wants to learn more about healthy coffee, but would rather receive text or video information, any URL / link can be sent to that person's email address-depending on which aspect they showed interest in. The prospective customer does have the opportunity to learn as much as they want once they visit the full CM system website [home page].

Meanwhile, the system sends 'follow-up emails' to remind the prospective customer of their initial interest in the product and/or opportunity. Each of the email messages encourages the prospect to re-visit the site and to contact the Distributor to learn more or try the products. During this time, I send my own email to the prospective customer to find out if they want to sample the product. NOTE: As you may know, it is getting more and more difficult for email messages to get through to their intended recipients because of over-zealous email filters; therefore, some or all of the emails from the CM system may end up in the persons 'junk mail' box instead. With that in mind, it is a good idea to phone the person, if they included their phone number, as soon as possible after they have initiated interest. This book will help you answer a lot of the questions most people ask initially.

Besides this system, I also personally use a facebook fanpage, traffic exchanges, list builders, widget ads, social media and VIP pages (video-search-engine-optimized pages) as well as creating informative, and sometimes humorous, YouTube videos. By layering and building upon these methods, over time, the Distributor that invests his/her time and effort in this manner, will have a better chance of being 'found' online whenever someone, especially in their local area, is conducting a search engine search on 'healthy coffee' or similar search terms [these are methods any business owner can use for any other type of business as well]. This may very well be how you came upon this book and the reason you are now reading it! If a Distributor shared this book with you, you should contact him / her after you've read through the information, request a sample, and ask to attend a CJM in your area. These methods can be utilized by any distributor. The CM system includes pre-recorded orientations, tutorials, and ads including sales letters and classified ads; offline & online marketing tools & information.

Other options any Distributor can use are:

- Create your own website
- Utilize Classified Ads
- Create YouTube videos

- **Utilize Social Media site such as Facebook and Twitter**
- **Online advertising sites – free and paid**

You may want to ask your chosen Distributor for sites that he/she uses to advertise online, and you can also search online via a search engine by typing 'Online Advertising' or 'Online Promotion'. Nowadays, there are several sites that offer free websites you can customize yourself, free classifieds, etc. The CM system training & support section includes video tutorials on copywriting, list building, blogging and much more.

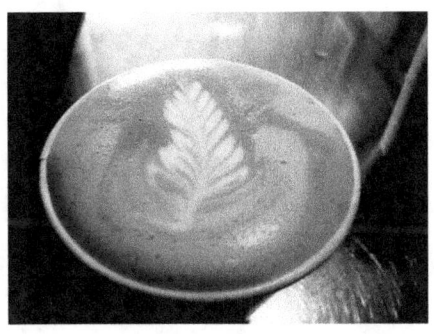

HOW DO I PROMOTE MY COFFEE PRODUCTS OFFLINE?

1. **Direct Mail such as postcards.**
2. **Magazine ads**
3. **Contact friends and family using the COFFEE SCRIPT**
4. **Inviting to CJMs**
5. **Promotional materials such as tee shirts, signs, bumper stickers, business cards [make sure you own a domain name that re-directs to your company replicated site, website, or blog, and one that re-directs to your favourite (and most compelling) lead capture page if you choose to use the CM system.**
6. **An 800 number with a pre-recorded message that [at the end] allows callers to**

leave their information so they can receive a sample and /or a callback or even an invite to a local event.

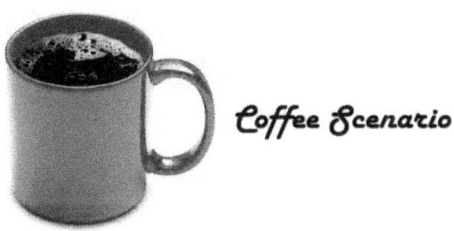

Coffee Scenario

COFFEE SCENARIO #8

Example COFFEE SCRIPT:

Hello first name! [make small talk here for a moment, and then get to the purpose of your call]. Listen first name, I only have a minute, but I wanted to tell you that I just started a healthy beverage company and I am launching it with 3 flavours of healthy coffee. Yes, that's right I said healthy coffee. First name, I need your help. I would like to have you as one of my first customers by buying some coffee from me. If you like the coffee I will show you how to get it at wholesale price, but if you don't like it, I will buy it back from you, and I will never ever ask you to buy anything from my company again.

Can I count on your support? [Tell them WHY you are doing this: why you need or want to earn extra income. If they launched a business, would you support them? Tell them so!]

They will ask how much does it cost and you tell them $34.00 box Retail (approximately), but if they end up liking it and wanting more, you will show them how to get it for $17.00 a box. ASK THEM: How many boxes do you want to buy??? Take the order, collect payment, and schedule the delivery. When you deliver the product(s), you may want to have a cup with them and show them an overview DVD presentation to learn how they can buy it wholesale. Ask them for their testimony. Don't forget to ask for referrals.

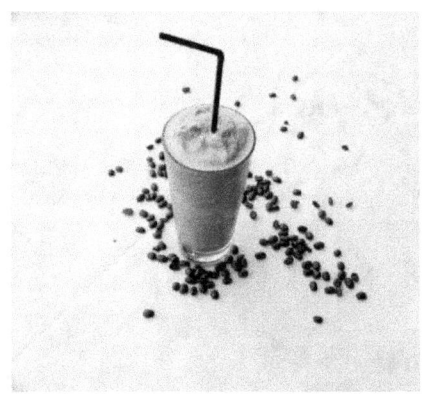

DO YOU HAVE A SALES LETTER I CAN USE TO GENERATE SALES?

Yes. The CM system sends a series of 'sales letters' via email that you can glean information from, and the system also has 'solo ads' and 'ppc [pay per click] ads'- think 'mini classified ads that are eye-catching and attention-grabbing'. Opt in [enter your name and email address] into a Distributor's CM system lead capture page, and save the series of emails you will receive. Study them to learn how best to craft your own sales letters.

Plus the COFFEE SCRIPT is a sort of verbal 'sales letter' too [ask your sponsor for the script!].

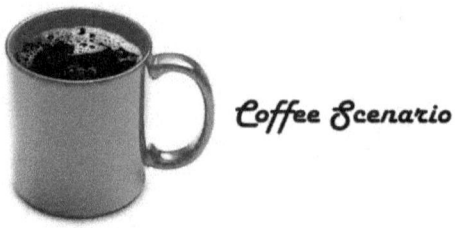

Coffee Scenario

COFFEE SCENARIO #9

A basic Sales Letter here:

If you're looking for success, and you're sick and tired of over hyped, over priced and underperforming products, then this may be your lucky day. If you are looking to grab a little extra income in these tough economic times, you may be surprised to know that there is a better way than trying to convince people to use some exotic juice or the latest miracle lotion or potion.

What if you were offering a product already used by 255 million people every day? I am not kidding when I say that if anyone tried to stop these people from consuming this product... things would get ugly, and fast!

Isn't it time you moved to the front of the line? Take a quick trip over to my website at 'your website link' and find out exactly how you can

position yourself between the 255 million people and the 9 billion dollars they spend every year.

Your Contact Info Here

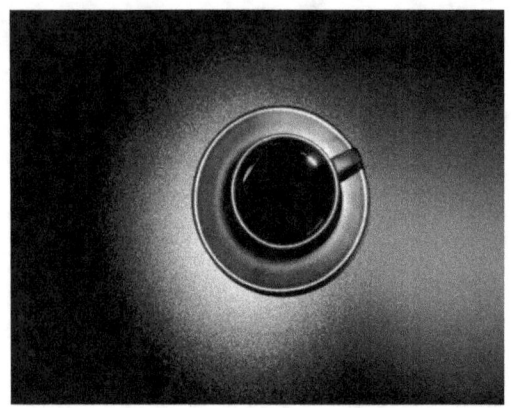

DO YOU HAVE CLASSIFIED ADS I CAN USE TO GENERATE SALES?

Yes. The CM system has classified ads you can use, or tweak a bit to make them your own. You may use them in print classifieds and online classifieds.

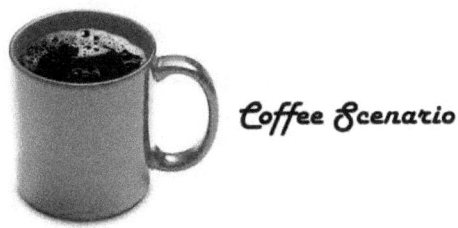

Coffee Scenario

COFFEE SCENARIO #10

A few Basic Classified Ads – for Online Placement:

The New Healthy Coffee Revolution
Pays You To Drink Coffee
www.yourwebsitehere.com

Be A Coffee Millionaire
255 Million Potential Customers
Ready To Buy From You
www.yourwebsitehere.com

Drink Starbucks Coffee?
Get The Same Bold Flavor and A
Huge Payday Just for Trying Ours
www.yourwebsitehere.com

Get Paid To Drink Coffee
Healthy Coffee Has Finally Arrived
www.yourwebsitehere.com

The World's Best Tasting Coffee
Get the amazing health benefits and
A healthy paycheck in your next cup
www.yourwebsitehere.com

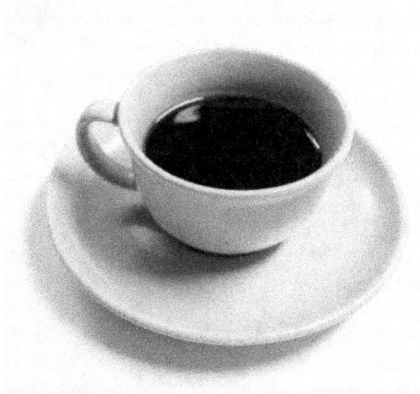

DO YOU HAVE A LIST OF PLACES I CAN ADVERTISE TO ONLINE?

Yes. The CM system has a listing of places you can place ads at, including free and paid methods. I personally use many online methods to advertise with [because my current physical condition limits my ability to 'get around']. Make sure to ask your chosen Distributor for places he/she utilizes to advertise online. There are many free and paid sites you can choose to advertise on. Do a search engine search for 'advertise online' too.

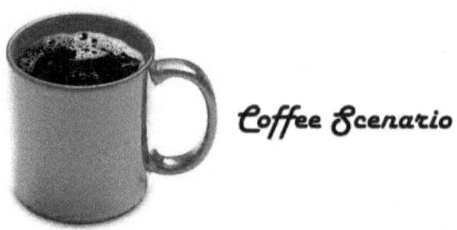

Coffee Scenario

COFFEE SCENARIO #11

A few Basic Classified Ads – for Offline [print] Placement:
Stop Paying for your Coffee
Let Your Coffee Pay You
Make Big Money With a Simple Plan
555 555 5555 or www.yourwebsitehere.com

Do You Like Coffee or Tea?
Do You Need More Money?
Watch This Coffee Video Now
www.yourwebsitehere.com

Tap Into A 9 Billion Dollar Market
255 Million Potential Customers and
Six Figure Income Potential in your First
Year. 555-555-5555 or
www.yourwebsitehere.com

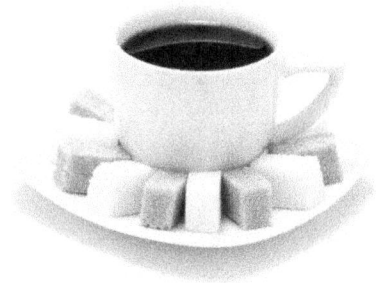

DO YOU HAVE A LIST OF PLACES I CAN USE TO ADVERTISE OFFLINE?

Yes. You can use [type these names individually into a search engine search online to find them] craigslist, backpage, thrifty nickel, and any magazines of the healthy sort. The CM system has a listing of places you can place offline advertising ads with. Don't be afraid to ask your chosen Distributor where he/she advertises offline and online. Because there are many places, free and paid, to promote your business with online, I highly recommend that you do both. Ask your chosen Distributor for specific ads to use as well. If he/she has flyers, postcards, signs, templates-ask for them. Tweak them to make them your own. Then get them out where everyone can learn about your coffee. See the Coffee Scenario ads I have in this book too.

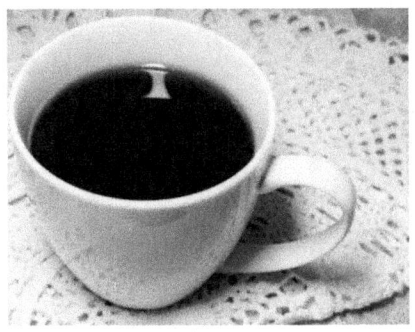

HOW DO I SHARE THIS PRODUCT WITH MY FRIENDS AND FAMILY?

Use the COFFEE SCRIPT to pre-sell your coffee at the launch of your business. Ask your sponsor for assistance with this method. Sample your product quickly to your first list of friends and family, and opportunity seekers that you personally know, so that you can start building your group of retail and wholesale customers. Invite them to your first CJMs as well-and ask them to share their personal experience with everyone attending.

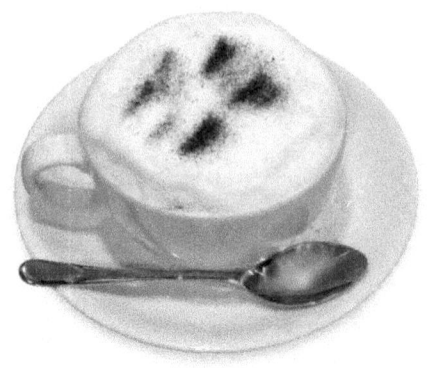

HOW DO I SHARE THIS PRODUCT WITH 'STRANGERS'?

Carry your sachets with you, make sure you have business cards or some contact info on the sachet so that when you meet people you want to share this with, any place, any time, you can hand them a sample and ask for their contact info so you can follow-up within 24 to 48 hours on how they liked the taste and how it made them feel. For those samplers that are interested: give them more information, invite them to a local CJM, or even do a one-on-one overview, etc.

You can also create a gift basket of samples (for example if you wanted to introduce this to an office group or fitness center) and brochures, or samples and Health News issues [each one with your complete contact info]. I recommend that you also include business cards and a note on how to mix properly, for best taste experience. Let them know you will follow up in one to two days. Follow-up, take orders, send more information, and invite coffee and tea lovers to CJMs, etc.

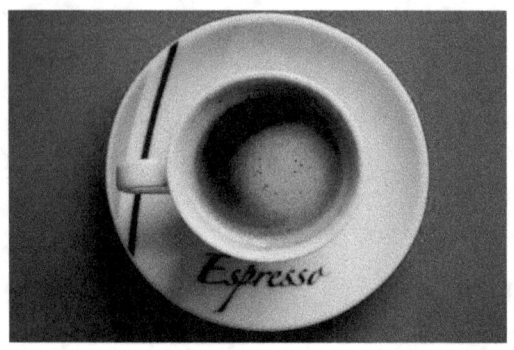

HOW MANY WAYS CAN I GET PAID TO DRINK AND SHARE THIS?

With this particular brand of healthy coffee, you can earn income seven different ways. Ask your sponsor for more information and details on this. There is also a Compensation Plan PDF when you log into your company provided website [along with many other documents and information sheets].

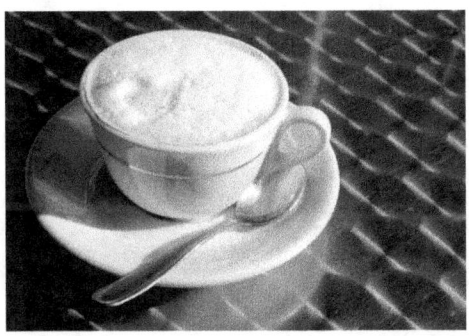

WHAT ARE THE 4 STEPS TO SUCCESS?

There are four steps you will want to follow for best results and to save time, money and energy on your part! Ask your sponsor for clarification. Basically:

1. Become a product of the product [consume the products, submit your own personal testimonial, setup autoship to be prepared for your own consumption, for sampling, for resale, etc].
2. Build a list of contacts as mentioned previously [50 people that know, like and trust you and 50 people that you know are open to opportunities to earn additional income]
3. Book Four CJMs [Schedule four mixers that you will host ASAP].

4. **Plug into the Proven Success System [Your chosen Distributor (your Sponsor) will give you all the details on trainings, events, calls, and online communities that will help you achieve your own goals].**

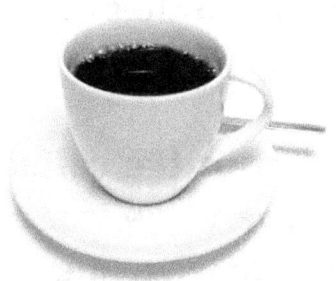

WHAT ARE THE 4 QUESTIONS?

The '4 Questions' is a simple way for you to remember how to share sachets of coffee, more efficiently. This is to see if the people you introduce it to will want to try it, and want to buy it. Let them decide, after they've experienced the taste and feel, what they want to do next. Here is what you ask, and the order in which you ask it in:

1. Do you or anyone you know drink coffee or tea at least occasionally?
2. How do you drink your coffee?
3. What brand do you like the best?

4. When was the last time [that company they like the best] sent you a check for drinking their coffee?

You then say 'Well, this is the coffee that pays you; I am happy to give you a free sample, but only if you promise to give me 2 pieces of information, would that be OK?'
If they say OK, get their contact information [best phone number to reach them and perhaps email address as well] and follow-up within 24 to 48 hours. If they say it is NOT OK, then thank them for their time and walk away with your sachets in hand.
For those that said 'OK', call them after a day or two, and ask if they liked the taste, and / or they noticed some type of benefit, and then let them know you can get more products for them. They will likely ask for pricing and quantity information.

Schedule a time to deliver their products after collecting payment. Or, simply send them to your company site [depending on location and relationship] to order.

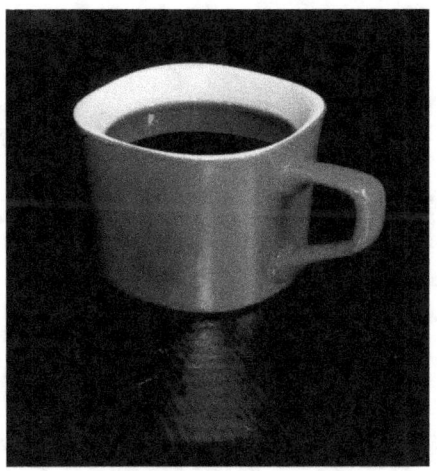

WHAT DO I DO NOW?

Simple. Make a Decision:

1. **Do Nothing.**
2. **Locate an Independent Distributor and request a sample.**
3. **Ask your chosen Distributor for a link to Watch an Overview presentation via Video, a phone number & PIN to Listen to a Live Overview Call, or better yet-meet directly with your chosen Distributor for one on one communication about this brand, and to answer your questions and concerns.**
4. **Buy Coffee or Products at Retail Price.**
5. **Buy Coffee or Products at Wholesale Price, as a Wholesale Customer.**

6. Become a Distributor and follow the system outlined above & with the assistance of your chosen Distributor, so that you can work towards getting whatever it is that you want to achieve by using Healthy Coffee as the vehicle to get you there.

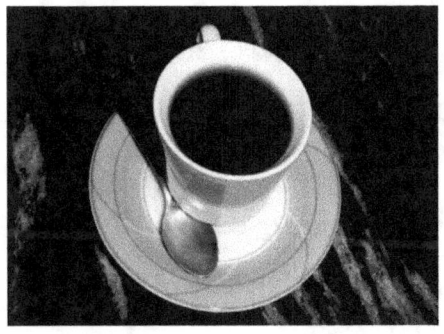

MY PERSONAL TESTIMONY

After 2 1/2 weeks of drinking this coffee, I noticed that my high blood pressure readings were much lower than before [they shot up sky-high after an auto accident, even after I was placed on prescription medication to lower it] . I kept drinking at least one cup a day not only because of the additional health benefits but because of the exquisite taste. I not only have noticed my lowered blood pressure, but also: less headaches & migraines. Over time I noticed my nails and hair looked healthier. My skin looks better. I am a calmer, happier person. Despite my physical injuries, I am able to manage the pain better, and I have more flexibility now. I firmly believe that if it weren't for my daily consumption of this product, I'd have to rely more heavily on prescription pain medications, and I'd probably not be able to 'get around' as much. Shortly after drinking my first cups, I noticed that I wasn't experiencing any of the 'usual' issues I had before with 'regular' coffee: nausea, burning stomach, caffeine jitters & crashes. Some of the allergens that affected me horribly are now non-existent. I also no longer have morning sugar cravings [I recall having to have some type of donut, pastry or sweet of some sort, for over 20 years, every single morning, to accompany my regular coffee!]. In my humble opinion, there is no better-tasting coffee on the Planet. For me, it is easy to share this brand of coffee simply because of the taste. But it is also a keeper because of the value and benefits it can bring into a person's life.

This coffee has changed my life completely and I am forever grateful to the person that decided to share it with me [my Sponsor whom I met online on a social media site, and after communicating for a couple of weeks, he asked me if I drank coffee, and if I would like to sample a new brand]. Because of the taste, my overall increase in my wellbeing, the high quality of the products, the affordable prices and much more, I will continue to consume this brand of healthy coffee.

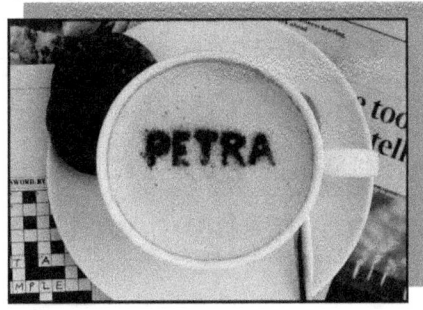

-Petra Ortiz

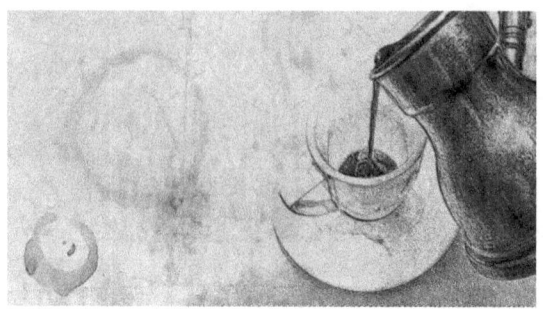

CONCLUSION

Thank you for reading my book. It means a lot to me that you took the time to do so. And I truly hope that it benefits you, or someone you care about, in some way. If you plan on becoming a Retail or Wholesale customer, you will not need to read the rest of the information I have written in this chapter.

For those of you that have read this far: this was meant to give you the 'big picture'; it is better for you to actually consult with an Independent Distributor for clarification, and, if you want, robust assistance in achieving your specific goals. Are you a good communicator? A good communicator helps people get what they want. Are you willing to help people and do you truly want to improve other people's quality of life? You will need to know what to say to people when you call them, when they place an order, when they ask for help and training. Besides learning how to communicate effectively, and especially if you decide that you want to share this brand of healthy coffee [whether to earn additional income or not] these are some traits you will want to have, and look for in others, that are seeking to have more time freedom and financial freedom: possess high self-esteem, are goal-driven, have an entrepreneurial spirit, are ready to act 'now', are mentally tough, are business-minded, decisive, and open-minded.

Are you willing to invest your time in learning how to set appointments, how to invite to a presentation, how to present, how to sponsor and train new people? If so, then you are on the right track for success. Stick with your chosen Distributor's suggestions and advice. It is in his/her best interest to help you succeed. And that's the best person to have in your corner any time. Learn how to be effective, so that you are self-motivated.

Thank you for reading this book. If the information provided in this book has helped you in any way, I'd surely like to hear about it [thank you!]. Now go and do what you feel is right for you. By the way, are you going to share what you've learned?

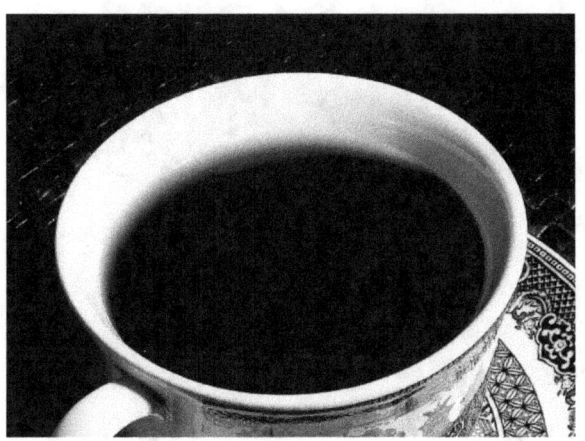

THE END

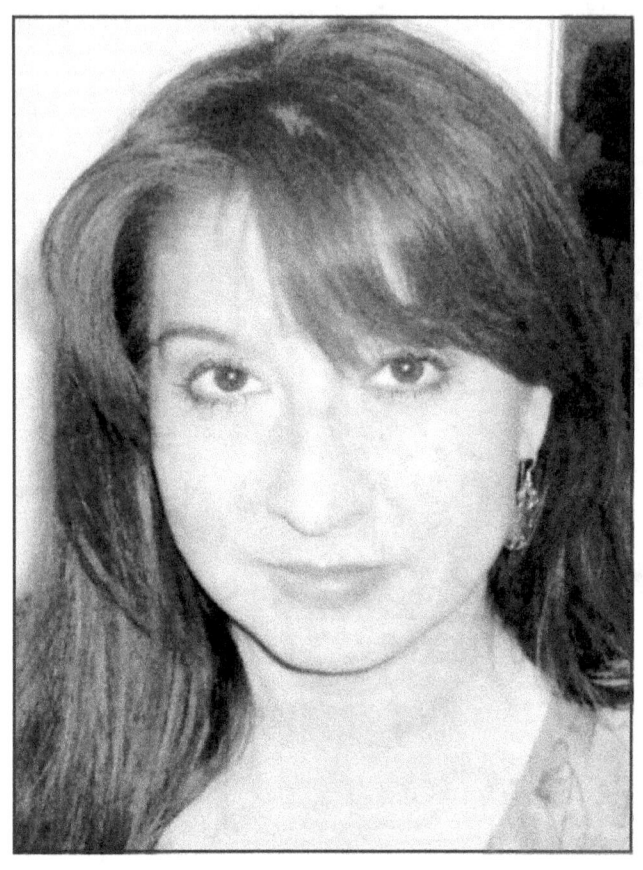

TO LEARN MORE ABOUT THE AUTHOR, PLEASE VISIT:
www.facebook.com/petralovescoffee

www.ingramcontent.com/pod-product-compliance
Lightning Source LLC
Chambersburg PA
CBHW070158290526
45789CB00002B/824